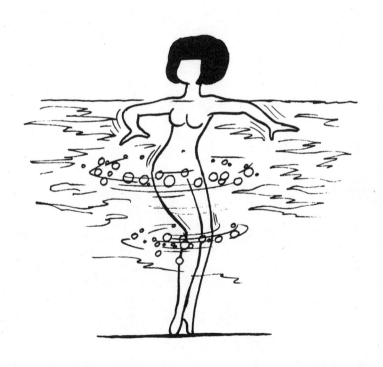

AQUA-RHYTHMICS

Exercises for the Swimming Pool

by ILSE NOLTE-HEURITSCH

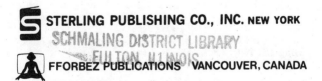

STERLING PUBLISHING CO., INC. NEW YORK

FFORBEZ PUBLICATIONS VANCOUVER, CANADA

OTHER BOOKS OF INTEREST

Better Roller Skating

Getting Started in Tennis

Golf Explained

Gymnastics

Handball Basics

Tumbling and Trampolining

Jazz Dance & Jazz Gymnastics

Front cover photo by Kelvin Mah
Drawings by Gerold Teigschl
Translated by Norma Wieland

Second Printing, 1979
Copyright © 1978 in United States by Sterling Publishing Co., Inc.
Two Park Avenue, New York, N.Y. 10016
Copyright © 1978 in Canada by Fforbez Enterprises Ltd.
Box 35340, Vancouver, B.C.
Original edition published in Germany under the title, "Aqua-Rhythmik,"
© 1977 by Falken Verlag, Niedernhausen/Taunus
Manufactured in the United States of America
All rights reserved
Library of Congress Catalog Card No.: 78-57782
Sterling ISBN 0-8069-4130-8 Trade
4132-4 Paper
4131-6 Library

Contents

A Personal Introduction 7
The Ideal Figure: A Big Problem 9
Water and How It Can Help You 12
   The Qualities of Water
Who Can Do Aqua-Rhythmics? 15
Aqua-Rhythmics: Where and How? 17
   The Swimming Pool . . . With or Without a Swim-
   suit . . . The Individual and the Group
The Basic Principles of Aqua-Rhythmics 19
   Varying the Rhythm . . . Varying the Direction . . .
   Varying the Movements
Arrangement of the Exercises 21
   The Basic Regimen . . . The Specialized Regimen
The Basic Regimen 23
   Swimming . . . Kicking . . . Treading Water . . . The
   Frog by the Wall . . . The Dancer . . . The Superkick
   . . . Swimming in Place . . . Scissors . . . The Shake
   . . . Jack-Knife . . . Bicycle . . . Frog in the Pool
The Refreshing Pause 50
The Special Regimen 52
   Posture . . . Exercises at the Wall and in the Middle of
   the Pool . . . Leg Circling (Standing Position) . . . Leg
   Circling (While Floating on Your Back) . . . Figure
   Eights . . . Floating Eights . . . Bent Circles and

Figure Eights . . . Arm Circling and Figure Eights . . .
Circles Galore . . . The Flipper . . . Fluttering . . . Flip
and Flutter . . . The Little Angel . . . Push and Swing
. . . The Stork Walk and the Stork Leap . . . The
Figurehead . . . Along the Wall . . . The Pendulum . . .
The Big Kick . . . The Bell . . . The Big Wave . . .
Horizontal . . . The Locomotive . . . The Water
Snake . . . The Twist . . . Jumping Jack . . . Spinning
Top . . . The Thriller . . . The Big Bell

Combinations and Inventions 92
How to Keep Your Good Figure 93
Index 94

A Personal Introduction

When I was 20 years old I was trim and slender, 5 foot 10 inches (175 cm) tall, and wore size 12 clothes. For 14 years my figure hardly changed at all. This marvellous situation did not have anything to do with any natural gift—it was directly related to my profession. I had studied gymnastics, rhythmics and dance and taught these subjects in Vienna. Later I had my own school and dance troupe. My job required so much energy that I couldn't possibly have a weight problem.

When I was 34 I changed my job and my life-style completely. There was no more daily training. Official receptions, cocktail parties and job-related dinner parties replaced it. As I became more successful and prosperous I hardly noticed the first few little extra pounds. But these few little pounds soon accumulated—and all in the wrong places, too. I got more and more comfortable and apathetic. Of course I didn't completely ignore the situation. I was constantly forcing myself to try various diets and when I was younger I could see that these attempts yielded some results. But they never lasted for very long. Staying slim required so much determination, exertion and sacrifice that it became harder and harder to keep in shape as the years passed.

Strangely enough, the most difficult thing for me to do was the one activity I'd been expert in—namely, gymnastics. By an heroic effort I managed to keep to a daily 15-minute training regimen, but exercises which had once come easily were beyond my strength now that I had put on weight. And when I did any jumping-in-place, my poor feet really protested. Real gymnastic leaps were now completely out of the question.

Soon I was more than 50 pounds (22 kilos) overweight and had other health problems which forced me to seek medical treatment. It was then that I first discovered underwater therapy which proved to be a successful curative as well as a wonderful way of developing and retaining a slim figure. This gave me the idea of adapting rhythmic exercises for the water, where even seriously overweight people could move more easily than they could on land. After I'd done a few of these exercises I was amazed at how much fun the whole thing was. All the unpleasant side effects encountered on dry land were gone—the sweating, exhaustion and sore muscles—yet the rolls of fat disappeared bit by bit. The specialized rhythmic exercises in the water were really even more effective than I'd expected.

At the same time I made some definite changes in my eating habits. I began eating wisely—and in smaller amounts—and still didn't go hungry. The combination of proper nutrition and exercise guarantees a good figure. After three months I could hardly believe the results. I had lost 44 pounds (20 kilos) and all from the right places, too! My skin felt firm and tingled with good health. I had my ideal figure back and would be able to keep it now.

My friends persuaded me to pass on my formula for success and so I taught them the various Aqua-Rhythmic exercises. The positive results I witnessed confirmed my method's effectiveness. This prompted me to write my experiences down so that other people could learn about the advantages of Aqua-Rhythmics. In this book you'll find both basic and specialized exercises. Make up your mind to give them a try—you won't regret it!

The Ideal Figure: A Big Problem

Gone are the good old days when rotund forms were compared to Rubens' paintings, when an overweight person was described as having a "stately figure." Today's ideal figure is slim. Being slim means that you don't have any extra weight to carry about and you can convert your energy into movement and activity—and thus into beauty, health, success and happiness, the dream of all overweight people.

However, our life-styles seem directly opposed to these goals and that's why obesity has become, in the literal meaning of the word, a very weighty problem nowadays. Through the achievements of civilization we have been provided with an increasingly easy life. Worse still, this easy life coupled with bad eating and drinking habits has actually become a status symbol. The results are shocking. A large number of people in our prosperous society suffer from obesity. This doesn't mean that we don't realize how this mode of living ruins our appearance, our success and our fun in life. But it's very hard to give up comfort and enjoyment. "If only we could buy an ideal figure," many people sigh, as their seams burst with their prosperity.

It's no wonder that the question, "How can I lose weight?" is more common today than ever before. Statistics show that every overweight person has tried to reduce at least once, if not several times. All overweight people agree that the slimming process must be as fast and as easy as possible. All kinds of reducing systems are promoted and the more sensational the promise of quick weight loss, the more people take note of them. But people usually can't keep up a mood of sacrifice for very long and they give up the tiring and uncomfortable effort after two or three weeks. If they have managed to keep going they're often tired and irritable. Their skin sags, making them look older than before. Sure, they've lost weight, but not always from the right places, and in addition they have to adjust their life-style in the future, too, to try to prevent regaining those lost pounds. It doesn't take long before they've reverted to their old ways.

However, there is a sensible way to lose weight: Aqua-Rhythmics. With this method you can get rid of excess pounds in all the right places, because it can be directed at specific areas. You won't merely lose weight, you'll get your good figure back—in fact, you can achieve your own personal ideal figure. Since no two people are exactly alike, a tall, heavy person, even when slim, has quite a different shape from a small, compact one. This fact should always be borne in mind. Many people have illusions about their appearance. How else could we explain the fact that so many people happily wear shorts or bikinis when their shapes aren't suited to them at all. The perfect figures that we see in magazines and films can give us misleading ideas. It doesn't do any harm, of course, to use these models as spurs to doing something about our own shapes, but to want our figures to be exactly like theirs can only lead to unhappiness and dissatisfaction. Each person has his or her limits and once you have achieved your optimal figure you should be satisfied with it and do all you can to retain it.

Each person has to decide for himself or herself how much weight to take off and where. Your scales will tell you the amount and only they can point out how far your own weight is above the average. You should consult them at least twice a week so that you can keep a continual check on all changes in your weight. Your clothes can suggest to you where your superfluous pounds are—but only the mirror can show them. That's why it's even more important than the scales when it comes to slimming, and so you should also consult it at least twice a week.

With the help of scales and a mirror you've answered the question of how much weight you have to lose and where you have to lose it. Now comes the really important question, "How am I going to do it? How can I attain my ideal figure?" The answer is: by letting the water help you!

Water and How It Can Help You

It really isn't necessary to tell you how beneficial water is, as we all have ample proof of its wonderful qualities. The doctors of ancient times knew about the healing properties of water and these are still demonstrated in modern pool therapy which has helped many seriously ill and incurable patients.

The right to make use of the wonderful power of water has not always belonged to doctors alone. In German-speaking countries we have the example of Pastor Kneipp. Sick and without hope, he experienced the curative effect of water on his own body and, deeply convinced of the value of his discovery, he helped many fellow sufferers in the same way. From these experiences he developed his own water cure which he promoted despite criticism and which he constantly practiced and preached. The accuracy of his beliefs has been proved by the fact that his cures are just as viable today as they were one hundred years ago. His methods, without modification, are still successfully applied today in Germany and Austria.

Very few people are aware of the healthful properties of water in this respect, probably because its curative aspects have always been used to help sick rather than healthy people. For most people water is something they use for sport and recreation. But if water can help so many sick people, think of how much more easily and rapidly it could help healthy people—and why not overweight people too? Let's make the water our helper and ally in our efforts to achieve an ideal figure. Let's concentrate especially on those underwater movements which lead to slimness, beauty and mobility of the body:

namely, Aqua-Rhythmics. They will reduce weight, prevent us from putting on weight and help us maintain a good figure.

The Qualities of Water

The buoyancy of water is particularly important. It frees you from your own weight and restores your freedom of movement. Your elasticity is effortlessly increased and you can easily perform exercises which you would find either impossible or incredibly strenuous on land.

A sense of security in the water is guaranteed by its buoyancy. This is of great psychological and physiological importance because it gives you the courage to move about and you can do all kinds of exercises in the water without the worry of injury. There's no need for overweight people—including overweight senior citizens—to be afraid that they might lose their balance or fall. The water will catch you. You can jump and hop around without overtaxing your poor feet. The water has three advantages: it gives you the courage to move about, it gives you the freedom to move about and it enables you to enjoy the sensation of doing just that! And all three of these things contribute to the success of Aqua-Rhythmics.

The resistance of the water has the effect of intensifying every exercise. As a result, the muscular tension and the speed at which you perform each movement has a greater effect on the body. The water resistance forces you to activate your muscles to the maximum degree and thus fatty padding has no chance of remaining for very long.

A refreshing massage is received with each movement in the water. This massage will be either gentle or vigorous depending on the strength of the movement. You can consciously achieve this effect by means of special exercises and by self-massage. Self-massage has a two-fold effect—it makes the hands slim and flexible while you manipulate fatty padding and cellulitis.

There are still more pleasant discoveries you can make in the water:

● After exercising in the water you feel you've done something and yet you don't have any sore muscles.

● You can feel the blood pleasantly pulsating throughout your body and you may feel a gentle tiredness, which is never exhaustion. After a short rest you're ready for new activity.

● If you're tense or tired when you get into the swimming pool, the exercises in the water make you bright and active again.

● Even the most strenuous exercises don't make you uncomfortable or sweaty.

Who Can Do Aqua-Rhythmics?

One of the advantages of Aqua-Rhythmics is that you can do the exercises (even if you're a non-swimmer) in any indoor pool regardless of the weather. This is especially important if you live in a region where the really warm days are numbered. Basically, anyone can take part in Aqua-Rhythmics. Unlike many other methods of reducing, Aqua-Rhythmics are not hazardous to your health—on the contrary, in fact. Even older people can perform Aqua-Rhythmic exercises without undue strain. Since the water supports your body, the danger of injury in a swimming pool is extremely low. Each person can perform the exercises as quickly as he or she likes and with as much energy as seems best. This makes Aqua-Rhythmics attractive even to senior citizens.

Aqua-Rhythmics are designed for the whole family. Take the example of a mother with a young child. On sunny days they might go to a playground where the mother sits on a bench and watches the child playing. The most she can do is read, chat or knit and what happens if the weather is bad? It would be a much better idea to go to a swimming pool where they would both get enjoyment—and benefits too. Aqua-Rhythmic exercises are like playing in the water, and children get a lot of fun out of that, especially if mother's there as a playmate. And isn't it true that often mother *and* child could both do with losing a bit of weight? Weekends and evenings father can join in Aqua-Rhythmics, too. After a hard day's work he can relax and recuperate in the water and the whole family is doing something together.

People who work behind a desk will quickly discover how good Aqua-Rhythmics are for the body. Arms and legs loosen up and muscles relax. The massage action of the water increases the circulation and frees you to move round any way you want. Thus Aqua-Rhythmics are really ideal for people who want to improve their figures without undue suffering. And you don't have to spend a lot of money to take advantage of them, either. Almost every town or city has a public swimming pool and admission costs very little. Everyone should try it out at least once!

Aqua-Rhythmics:
Where and How?

The Swimming Pool

What do you need if you're going to take up Aqua-Rhythmics? If you have your own swimming pool then you are very lucky. You can do the exercises every day or at least every two days. Most people will use public swimming pools, pools in youth clubs and health spas and—on holiday, for example—hotel swimming pools. Many new housing complexes have community pools.

The pool must fulfil the following requirements for Aqua-Rhythmics:

● You have to be able to stand up in it since you need the bottom under your feet for many exercises and it also makes you feel safer. The water should come up to your neck—otherwise the exercises will not make much sense. Your well-padded areas should be massaged by the water and not by the air.

● You have to be able to hold on to the edge of the pool without difficulty. You need this support for many of these exercises.

● The water should be at a comfortable temperature. You will stay in the pool for up to twenty minutes and you don't want to get chilled. If the water temperature is just right it doesn't matter what the weather is like outside.

Most pools fulfil these three basic requirements so it should not be hard to find a suitable place to practice Aqua-Rhythmics. The swimming pool of the future will be a real "slimming" pool with various apparatus in the water and music to accompany the exercises. You could vary the Aqua-Rhythmic exercises very nicely if you had a ladder in the water and a swing suspended over it. But even a ladder at the edge of the pool, the steps or the corner of the pool itself can be used to vary the exercises. That way Aqua-Rhythmics are even more fun and that makes them all the more effective.

With or Without a Swimsuit

We can compare the effect of the water to that of the sun. The sun only tans the portions of skin that are exposed to it. In the same way the massage action of the water works most powerfully on a nude body. However, very few people have their own pool, and water massage also works well if you wear a bikini or swim trunks. Very overweight women will probably start with a one-piece swimsuit, but with the help of Aqua-Rhythmics they will soon want to show off their figure and will be able to wear a two-piece suit. People who own their own pool or who have the opportunity to swim in the nude should certainly take advantage of it.

The Individual and the Group

Of course you will want to try out your exercises alone at first. Find a quiet place in the pool where you will not be in anyone's way and where no one can bother you. You will only need a small amount of space for most of the exercises. And the water is very discreet, too! If you are not able to do everything perfectly to begin with, no one will know. Later, however, it is a good idea to have an exercise partner or a small mixed exercise group. Then people are more likely to continue going to the pool on a regular basis, and they will also try harder because they can compare their progress with others.

You should not go about Aqua-Rhythmics in deadly earnest; it should be an enjoyable social event. Once you have mastered some of the basic exercises you can have a pleasant chat with your friends while you do them.

The Basic Principles of Aqua-Rhythmics

It's true in Aqua-Rhythmics that even the exercises which you don't perform perfectly at the beginning can often help you to lose weight. Once you know that, you don't have to feel constrained by the notion that you're only successful if you achieve perfection through hard work. The movements themselves and the fun you have doing them are more important than perfection. Once you're assured of that you can go ahead and do the exercises according to your abilities and your moods.

Rhythm and variations in direction and movement are especially important in Aqua-Rhythmics. If you always swim round at the same comfortable speed, for example, that is of course quite healthy—but you won't lose any weight that way. If you did all the exercises on one side, that would lead to one-sided muscular build-up which has neither a slimming nor esthetic effect. The more a movement lends itself to directional variation, the more effective it will be in making you slim and flexible.

Varying the Rhythm

One of the most important things in all exercises is the ability to vary the rhythm. That's actually why we call it "Aqua-Rhythmics" and not "water gymnastics." Each individual exercise is only really effective because of the variation of tensed and relaxed movements and because of changes in the tempo of the exercise. Here's how it works in practice:

• First of all, quite instinctively, you try to take the path of least resistance in performing an exercise so you can become completely familiar with it. You do it gently and loosely rather than rigidly. This mode we'll call "leisurely."

• Next you perform the same exercise exerting the greatest muscular tension against the resistance of the water. You have performed the exercise "energetically."

• Finally, you do the same exercise at double the speed. This pace we'll call "rapidly."

This constant variation from leisurely to energetically to rapidly is the secret of the new approach. The variations in rhythm are complemented and extended by variations in the movements themselves.

Varying the Direction

The direction of each exercise is determined by the aim and the aim is to get rid of all our unwanted rolls of fat. It is variation which determines whether you attack them directly or indirectly.

Varying the Movements

The human body is quite mobile in water so the exercises can be as varied as possible. We're always thinking, "How can I modify this exercise? For example, shall I do it with only my arms or only my legs? Or shall I use both together? Or maybe I can alternate, first arms, then legs."

If you think up variations in each movement along with variations in tempo and direction, then you won't get bored in the pool. You can take one movement and set up a whole regimen of variations on it.

Arrangement of the Exercises

You can't take this book into the water with you so the order as well as the names of the exercises have to be easy to remember.

Aqua-Rhythmics is divided into a basic regimen and a specialized regimen. Once you have mastered the basic exercises you should move the way *you* want to and try out any new combinations you like.

The Basic Regimen

The basic regimen is set up in such a way that your whole body gets a workout in the space of twenty minutes, and these exercises are aimed at all the critical areas. Although each person has his or her individual fat spots, most overweight people are thickly padded in the same places—thighs, abdomen, hips, and buttocks—and our basic exercises are aimed at these spots. You should repeat them as often as you need to master them completely. Only by doing the exercises in the basic regimen can you expect any decisive change in your figure.

The Specialized Regimen

You can only try a specialized exercise after you've worked your way through the entire basic regimen, and the complete basic regimen must remain as a prelude to any specialized one you undertake.

Here's how the specialized regimen works:

● You choose any exercise you like from the specialized regimen.

● You practice this specialized exercise until you master it. You can then add it to your standard repertoire of exercises.

● Then you can try a second and then a third specialized exercise and so on.

The Basic Regimen

Let's start with the basic regimen. It consists altogether of twelve basic exercise themes which you repeat until you know them perfectly. They are your fixed number of exercises and with their help you can really improve your figure. It doesn't matter what muscles you move when you do these exercises, the only thing that interests you is the effect they have on your well-padded areas.

Swimming

If you can swim, you should swim a few widths of the pool at a leisurely pace before you begin the Aqua-Rhythmics themselves. If you can't swim, don't worry, it isn't absolutely necessary for an effective Aqua-Rhythmics regimen. Just skip this exercise—none of the others demands any swimming ability.

Exercises:
1. Swim a certain distance, eight strokes, easily and loosely.
2. Now do eight strokes energetically.
3. Keep swimming and this time do eight strokes rapidly.

Note:
Just by varying from energetically to rapidly you've already got a completely new sensation of swimming.

Benefits:
When you swim the way you usually do, with the same calm, measured body movements, you only produce a sense of well-being. When you vary the force and tempo of the strokes, however, you're really starting to attack those first little rolls of fat.

Kicking

This is a movement we've all been able to do without practice since we were babies. Kicking is very good for the body, especially when it's done in the water.

Exercises :

1. Stand with your back to the wall of the pool and hold onto the pool rail at shoulder height, bending your arms slightly. Then, holding onto the rail, let yourself float in the water. Now kick to your heart's content until you're warm, eight times leisurely, eight times energetically, and eight times rapidly. (See Illus. 1.)
2. Turn round and lie on your stomach in the water. Holding on, and with arms slightly bent, kick as you did before, eight times leisurely, then eight times energetically, and eight times rapidly.

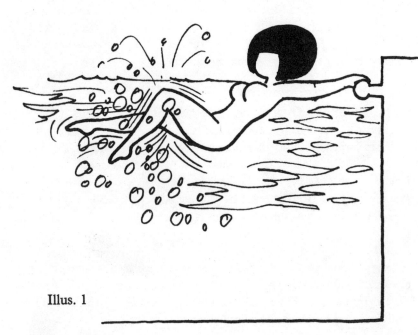

Illus. 1

You will have noticed that thrust and speed have different effects on your movements. Since the capacity for beginners differs in many respects, you will have to decide for yourself how many different exercises you will want to do.

Benefits:

The forward movement of the legs provides a good massage for your stomach and thighs and the backwards movement does the same for buttocks and thighs. You'll also get the feeling that the massage action of this exercise gets the useless fat moving.

The following three exercises come under the theme of "Knees Up." Here we'll do knee-raising variations—first one knee at a time. then left and right alternately, and then both knees together. When we combine these movements with variations from leisurely to energetically to rapidly, this produces eighteen different movements which benefit abdomen, hips, and buttocks. We'll begin by treading water which, when performed towards the side, gives us the "Frog by the Wall" (see page 29), and towards the back the "Dancer" (see page 31).

Treading Water

Starting Position:

Face the side of the pool and grasp the edge or handrail. Stretch your arms out loosely. Your legs should be together and comfortably straight.

Warm-Up:

1. Stand on your left leg on your tiptoes. Draw your right knee up towards your chest and lower it again to the starting position. Do this three times leisurely, three times energetically and three times rapidly. (In the last movements you will have trouble getting your foot back on the bottom.)

2. Repeat the same movements, this time raising your left leg. (See Illus. 2, 3, 4.)
3. Now raise both knees together towards your chest and then push your feet back towards the bottom of the pool. Do this four times leisurely, four times energetically and four times rapidly. (See Illus. 5.)

Exercise:

Standing in one spot, raise your legs alternately (first left and then right) so that you are "treading" water. Repeat eight times leisurely, eight times energetically and eight times rapidly. (See Illus. 6.)

Note:

You can feel the different effects of the variations on abdomen and legs. Optically the energetic movements will appear bigger than the rapid ones.

Benefits:

Treading water works on abdomen and thighs as well as calves, ankles and knees (especially when performed at double speed—"rapidly").

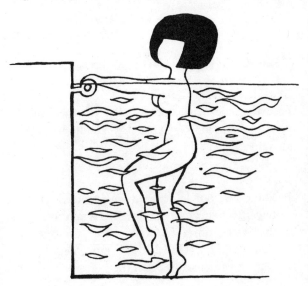

Illus. 2

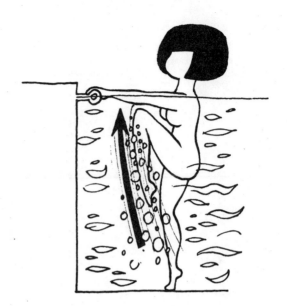

Illus. 3

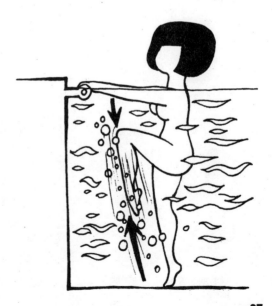

Illus. 4

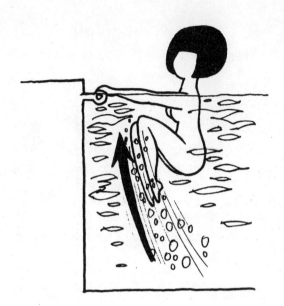

Illus. 5

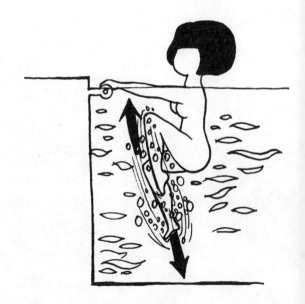

Illus. 6

The Frog by the Wall

The direction of the movement is now towards the side.

Starting Position:
As for "Treading Water."

Warm-Up:
1. Raise the right knee towards the side and push it down again. Repeat four times leisurely, four times energetically and four times rapidly. (See Illus. 7.)
2. Repeat the exercise with the left knee.
3. Now alternate the right and left knees, four times leisurely, four times energetically and four times rapidly. (See Illus. 8.)

Exercise:
Beginning in the same starting position, turn both knees outwards and draw them up at the same time. Repeat four times leisurely, four times energetical!y, and four times rapidly. (See Illus. 9.)

Benefits:
By changing the direction of the exercise you're now working on hips and legs.

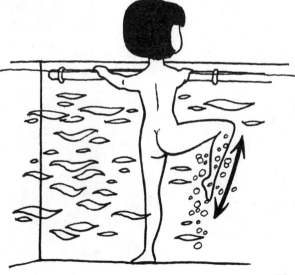

Illus. 7

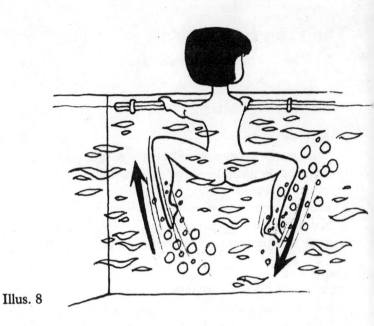

Illus. 8

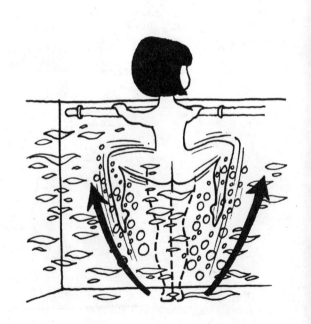

Illus. 9

The Dancer

Starting Position:
Same as for "Treading Water" (see page 25) and "Frog by the Wall" (see page 29).

Warm-Up:
1. Stand on your tiptoes and kick your left heel up behind you. Repeat four times leisurely, four times energetically, and four times rapidly. (See Illus. 10.)
2. Do the same thing with your right heel.
3. Now kick each heel behind you, alternating from left to right each time. Repeat four times leisurely, four times energetically, and four times rapidly. (See Illus. 11.)

Exercise:
Beginning in the same starting position, kick up both heels behind you simultaneously. Repeat four times leisurely, four times energetically, and four times rapidly. (See Illus. 12.)

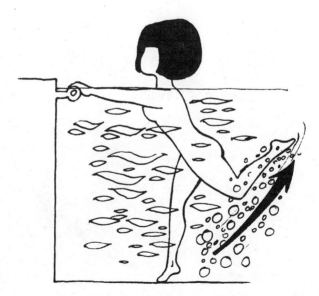

Illus. 10

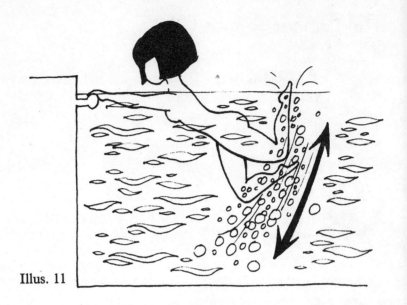

Illus. 11

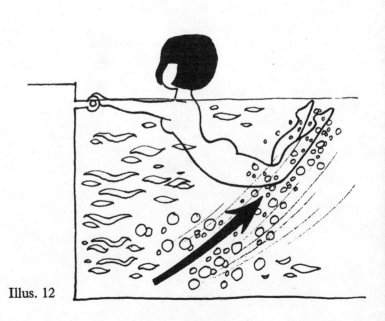

Illus. 12

Benefits:
By varying the direction you're able to concentrate on buttocks, back and thighs. To loosen up, shake your arms and legs.

Note:
Only a dancer could perform this exercise on land, but in the water it's quite easy.

We can invent other exercises which come under the theme of "Knees Up." For example, when you're "Treading Water" (see page 25) you can turn your body from the waist down. This will help you get a slim waistline. By adapting exercises in this way you can make them fit your own personal needs.

The Superkick

In this exercise you change the direction of your whole body and lie in the water, first on your back and then on your stomach. Hold onto the rail or the edge of the pool while you do this. You could now repeat all the steps of the previous exercise with different effect, of course. But instead we'll find another very effective exercise which is also fun to do.

Exercise:
1. Lie on your back in the water. Draw both legs together up towards your stomach and then stretch them out again. Repeat four times leisurely, four times energetically, and four times rapidly. (See Illus. 13.)
2. Turn round and lie on your stomach. Draw both legs up towards your stomach and stretch them out again. Repeat four times leisurely, four times energetically, and four times rapidly.
3. Now lie on your back again and alternately draw your left leg and then your right leg towards your stomach. Then both legs together. Repeat four times leisurely, four times energetically, and four times rapidly.

Benefits:

This exercise is aimed especially at the abdomen, and also at the stomach and thighs.

Now shake your arms, hands, legs, and feet again. Do this energetically at your own speed.

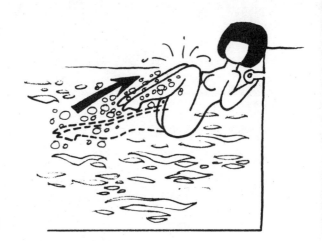

Illus. 13

Swimming in Place

Now you can turn your attention to your arms and upper body.

Warm-Up:

1. Stand with the edge of the pool to your left. Hold on with your left hand and stretch out your right arm sideways. Turn your right palm downwards, tense your arm and pull it downwards towards your side again. In other words, push the water towards your body. Repeat eight times leisurely, eight times energetically, and eight times rapidly.

2. Now do the same exercise with the other arm. Stand with the pool edge to your right, hold on with your right hand and stretch out your left arm. Now push the water towards you with your left arm. Repeat eight times leisurely, eight times energetically, and eight times rapidly.

3. Move away from the wall. With feet apart on the bottom, stand on your tiptoes and do the same exercise using both arms at once. (See Illus. 14.)

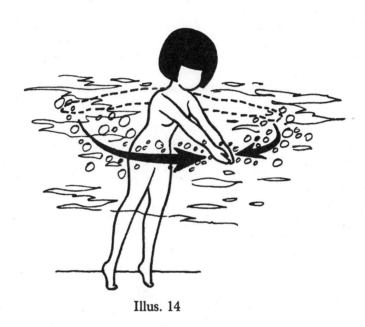

Illus. 14

Exercise:
1. Move away from the wall so you can stand freely.
2. Let yourself float in the pool and repeat the arm exercises described in the warm-up. These movements are the arm movements for the "Butterfly Stroke." Now do the "Frog Kick." That is to say, make the same movements with your legs as you are making with your arms. By using these countermovements of arms and legs, you are now swimming in place. Repeat eight times leisurely, eight times energetically, and eight times rapidly. (See Illus. 15.)

Note:
Non-swimmers can swim in place by doing warm-up exercises 1 and 2 with one hand on the rail. The other hand and arm perform the movements. You can "swim" with your right arm and right leg and your left leg will be very close to the bottom of the pool. Then hold on with your right hand and "swim" with your left arm and leg.

If, as a non-swimmer, you are really afraid to take your feet off the bottom, then simply repeat the two warm-ups.

Benefits:
The warm-ups work on arms, shoulders and chest.
Warm-up 3 is excellent as a breathing exercise, by the way. The actual exercise itself is good for the whole body.

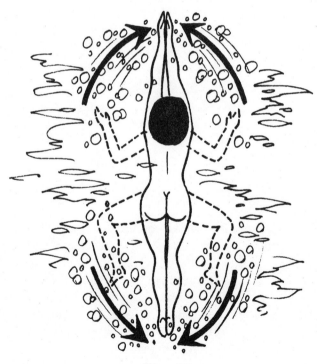

Illus. 15

Scissors

From the name alone you can envision what kind of leg exercise this is.

Warm-Up:
1. Stand with the pool rail to your left and hold on with your left hand. Stretch your right arm out in front of you at shoulder level. Now swing your right leg forwards as far as you can, trying for the surface of the water, then return to starting position. Keep your leg as straight as possible and put a good deal of energy into the upwards swing. Repeat the movement four times leisurely, four times energetically, and four times rapidly.
2. Now repeat the process with the other leg. Stand with the pool rail to your right, hold on with your right hand, stretch out your left arm in front of you and swing your left leg up towards the surface of the water and then back to starting position. Repeat four times leisurely, four times energetically, and four times rapidly. (See Illus. 16.)

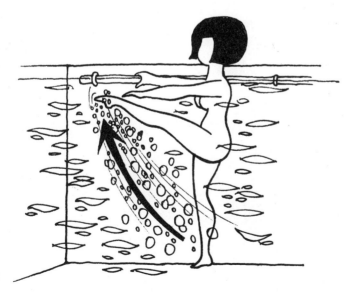

Illus. 16

3. Next you perform the same exercise sideways. (See Illus. 17.)
4. Do the same exercise, this time swinging your leg out behind you, rising onto your toes as you do so. (See Illus. 18.)
5. Stand once again with the pool rail on your left and hold on with your left hand. Stretch your right hand out in front of you at shoulder height. Without bending your knees, swing your right leg forwards as far as you can, but this time put more energy into the return swing as you force your leg back down to the starting position. Repeat four times leisurely, four times energetically, and four times rapidly.
6. Stand with the pool rail on your right and hold on with your right hand. Stretch your left arm out in front of you at shoulder height and, standing on your tiptoes, swing your left leg forwards, trying for the surface of the water, and then backwards. Again, you should put you energy into the return swing. Repeat four times leisurely, four times energetically, and four times rapidly. (See Illus. 19.)

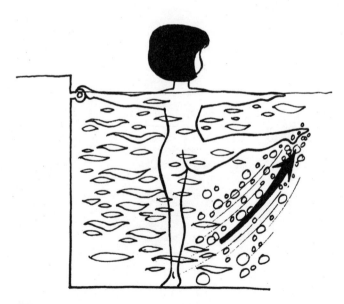

Illus. 17

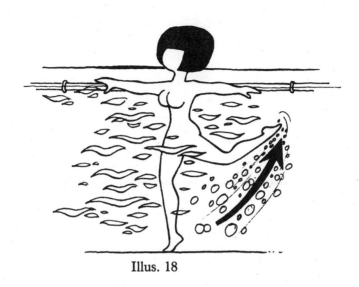

Illus. 18

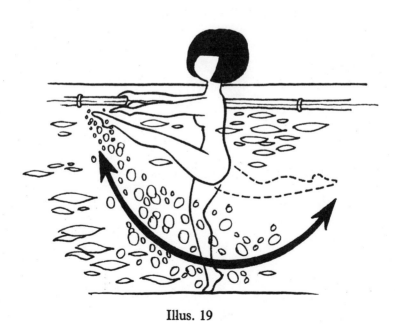

Illus. 19

Benefits:

Warm-up exercises 1 and 2 are aimed at the abdomen and thighs.
Exercise 3 aims at the hips and legs, exercises 4, 5 and 6 at the
buttocks and back. In addition, exercises 5 and 6 are good for the
abdomen and thighs. All the exercises provide a good massage for
the calves and waist.

Exercise:

With your back to the wall, hold onto the rail behind you with both
hands. Let your body float, relaxed, on the water. Both your arms
and your body should be straight.

1. Swing your outstretched legs up and down one after the other in
   quick succession (just like the movements of a scissors or the
   kick you use in the back stroke). Make the movements as wide as
   possible. Repeat four times leisurely, four times energetically, and
   four times rapidly. (See Illus. 20.)

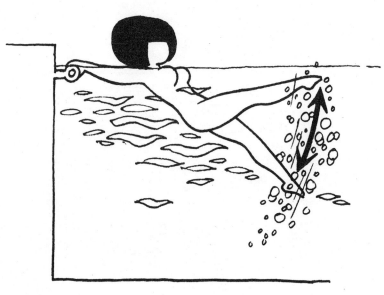

Illus. 20

2. Turn over and do the same exercise, this time lying on your stomach. Repeat four times leisurely, four times energetically, and four times rapidly.

Note:
This exercise is especially effective because it can be performed in so many different positions.

Benefits:
The upwards swing of the "Scissors" is good for abdomen and legs, the backwards swing is good for buttocks and back. It's hard to make a sharp distinction between the effects of this exercise when performed in the various positions.

The Shake

This exercise involves "shaking" your abdomen and hips.

Exercise:
1. Face the edge of the pool, both hands on the rail. Stand on the toes of your left foot and raise your right leg slightly sideways, without bending the knee. Now swing your abdomen in a full circle, first out towards the left, then back and round and out towards the front. Your upper body should move as little as possible. Do four circles leisurely, four energetically, and four rapidly. (See Illus. 21.)
2. Change legs and perform the same exercise in the opposite direction. Do four circles leisurely, four energetically, and four rapidly.
3. Now put your legs together and stand on your toes. Bend your knees a little and draw a full circle with your abdomen first starting out towards the left and then towards the right, alternating each time. Do eight circles leisurely, eight energetically, and eight rapidly.

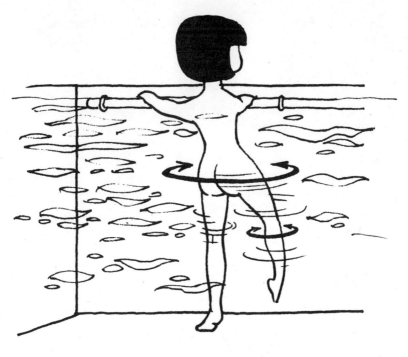

Illus. 21

Note:
This is a simple and very effective exercise and you really begin to feel the effects of it when you do it "rapidly." Then you've got all the well-padded areas moving and at the same time are giving yourself a first-class massage.

Benefits:
In addition to buttocks, hips, and abdomen, this exercise is also good for your waist.

Jack-Knife

Everyone takes great pleasure in jumping in the water, and it's also a very effective exercise. That's why we now move to the middle of the pool to try all kinds of jumping exercises. These jumps are the preparation for the "Jack-Knife."

Warm-Up:
1. Move to the middle of the pool. Stand on your tiptoes with your legs together, stretch your arms out sideways, rest them on the water—and jump!
2. At every second jump, swing your arms and legs forwards together. Do the whole thing eight times. With a little practice you'll be able to make your arms and legs touch. (See Illus. 22.)

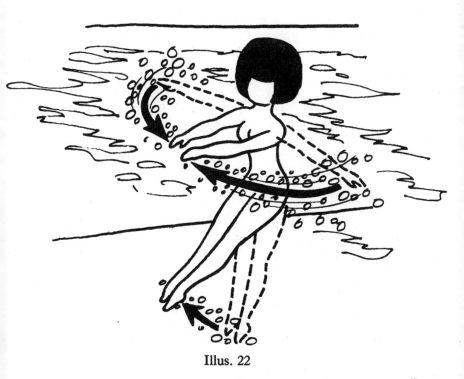

Illus. 22

Exercise:
1. Same starting position as for the warm-up.
2. This time don't jump up and down, but push off powerfully from the bottom with both feet and bend your body forwards so that, if possible, you touch your toes with your fingertips. This exercise will push you backwards in the water. (See Illus. 23.)

Note:
Make sure the area behind you is clear because with this exercise you can move about, rear-end first, all over the pool.

Benefits:
No padding can withstand this assault—especially not on the abdomen. At the same time your whole body, especially your arms and legs, is given a good workout.

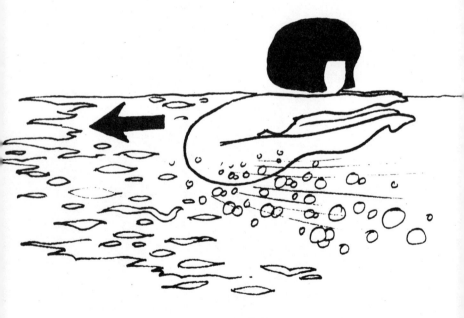

Illus. 23

Bicycle

Bicycling is something we're all familiar with and it's also a very good exercise.

Warm-Up:

1. Standing on your tiptoes, with the edge of the pool on your left and holding onto the rail with your left hand, raise your right knee and then straighten your leg out in front of you. Keeping your leg straight, push it back down to the starting position. Repeat four times leisurely, four times energetically, and four times rapidly.
2. Turn round and perform the same exercise with the other leg. Repeat four times leisurely, four times energetically, and four times rapidly. (See Illus. 24.)

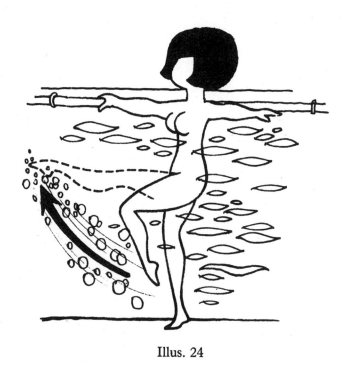

Illus. 24

3. Now do the same exercise, moving your legs out towards the back. Repeat four times leisurely, four times energetically, and four times rapidly. (See Illus. 25.)

Exercise:
1. Now, as you did for the "Scissors" exercise (see page 37), stand with the edge of the pool behind you. Hold onto the rail and, letting your body float on the water, pedal with your legs. Bicycle this way eight times leisurely, eight times energetically, and eight times rapidly.
2. Make use of the freedom of movement you have in the water and really stretch as you bicycle and, if possible, include your abdomen in the movements. Repeat eight times energetically and eight times rapidly.
3. Now pull up both knees together and then stretch your legs out. Do this four times leisurely.
4. Pull up both knees again and stretch your legs but this time use your abdomen and thrust yourself forwards like a wave. Repeat four times energetically and four times rapidly.

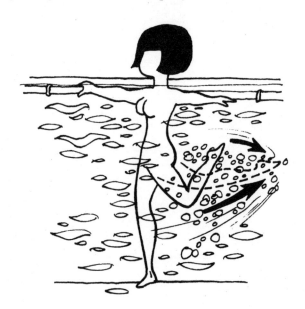

Illus. 25

Benefits:
The warm-up is good for feet, calves and thighs, the exercise itself for abdomen and thighs.

Variation 1:
Turn your abdomen towards the left and bicycle with your right leg making a big circle towards the left in front of you. Then turn your abdomen towards the right and bicycle with your left leg making a circle towards the right. Repeat eight times leisurely, eight times rapidly and then, alternating from left to right, perform the exercise eight times energetically. (See Illus. 26.)

Benefits:
This exercise makes your waist more flexible and also works on your abdomen.

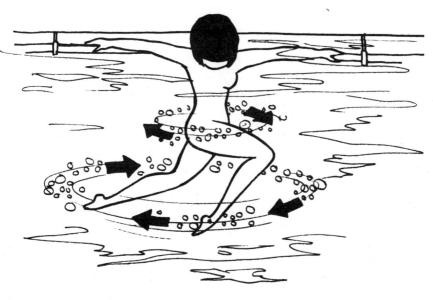

Illus. 26

Variation 2:
Lie on your stomach in the water and bicycle, but backwards; that is, stretch your leg out behind you and then pull your knee forwards as far as possible towards your stomach. Alternate with left and right legs.

Benefits:
Legs, abdomen, buttocks, hips and waist all are put to work when you do this exercise.

Frog in the Pool

To round out the basic regimen, find a spot in the middle of the pool. You've already practiced "Frog by the Wall" (see page 29), and can do it without any trouble. "Frog in the Pool" is the same exercise but without holding onto the rail.

Exercise:
1. Stretch your arms out sideways and let them rest on the water. Jump as forcefully as you can, pushing your knees out to the side. In this jump try to pull your knees up as far as possible.

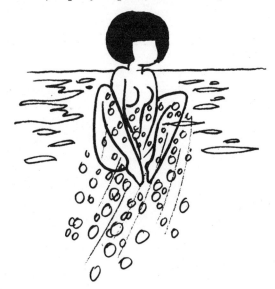

Illus. 27

2. At the same time, try to touch the soles of your feet with your hands. Jump four times energetically. (See Illus. 27.)

Benefits:
Good for thighs and hips as well as for arms and legs.

Variation:
You've already practiced this variation by the wall, too.
1. Jump forcefully, this time keeping your knees together and pulling them up to your chest with each leap.
2. At the same time, try to clap your hands together under your legs as you jump. Repeat four times energetically. (See Illus. 28.)

Benefits:
Works on the abdomen as well as on the arms and legs.

Note:
To finish up, do both exercises alternately. Only when you've got rid of all your rolls of fat will you be able to do the exercise perfectly.

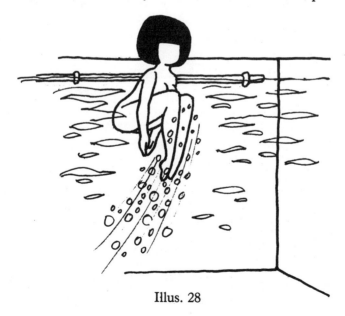

Illus. 28

The Refreshing Pause

Now it is time to leave the pool and take a well-deserved rest for half an hour. You should lie down for a while since everyone relaxes best in this position.

Remember that deep breathing is as important while resting as it is in all of the exercises. Of course, you're a little tired at this stage—but it is a relaxed tiredness. It does not matter if you have not managed to do all the exercises perfectly. The pleasure that comes from moving your body is more important than perfection. And you've certainly given your body a boost: your blood is pulsing, your circulation is quickened, and your lymphatic system is set in motion. You've shaken up your fatty cells and have started the breakdown process; they won't be able to resist your attacks for long.

The main benefit you should get from these exercises is the discovery that you are becoming more flexible—that shows you're making the right movements. But these encouraging thoughts should be translated into action right away: you can repeat the various exercises according to your preference—the ones you enjoyed most, the ones which had the most direct effect on your fatty areas, the ones you found the most difficult, or you can simply repeat all of them in the order in which you learned them. There are no limits to the ways you can practice and vary these exercises—it all depends on the way you feel.

You should have mastered the basic regimen in three to six weeks, depending on how eager and demanding you have been. At this point you'll be able to see the difference in your clothes: things that were too tight now fit loosely and you'll be astonished at your reflection in the mirror!

You look great—not just because you've lost some weight but because your muscles are taut, your posture has improved and there's a spring in your step. You've also gained self-confidence and that carries over into all your activities. You're now ready to devote yourself to the special exercises.

The Special Regimen

Having a good figure does not depend just on losing weight. Proportion and posture are also important. You can use the special exercises to attack those stubborn areas of fat which unbalance your figure.

The best way to start is to read through the entire special regimen. Then you can choose the exercises that will benefit your problem areas. Of course, you can also do all the exercises in the water first and then decide which ones have the greatest effect on your unwanted fat. There is one essential difference between this and the basic regimen: here you do each exercise until you have mastered it before you can move on to the next one. Remember that you must complete the entire basic regimen before you do any special exercises.

You've already learned from the basic regimen how the direction of an exercise determines the effect it will have. Here's a basic guide you can use: forward movements benefit abdomen and thighs, backwards movements benefit buttocks and back, sideward movements are good for hips and thighs and turning movements benefit the waist.

Alternations in tempo from "energetically" to "rapidly" determine how much of an effect an exercise will have. With this information at your fingertips you can now vary the special exercises quite easily. Just remember your motto in the water is "Do your own thing."

Posture

Good posture contributes a lot to a slender appearance. You've already done a great deal for your posture in the basic regimen, but now you should concentrate on doing each exercise carefully and beautifully.

Proper posture depends on your abdomen and upper body. Even the most beautiful figure won't help if you have rounded, hunched shoulders. This often leads to other problems—fatty padding at the back of the neck, spinal curvature and protruding abdomen. Since most of us unfortunately have to spend a large part of our day in a sitting position, the upper half of our bodies is much more visible than the lower half. That is why we've included special exercises for arms, shoulders and chest so that you can have a slender, mobile upper body.

These exercises should also encourage you to pay attention to the way you stand and sit in general, especially if you have a desk job. Concentrate on maintaining good posture while you're doing these exercises—especially the ones you do near the wall of the pool. Don't grasp the rail so tightly that you tense your shoulders or arms. Every now and then you should stop, take your hands off the rail and give them a good shake. A good way to test yourself is to stop suddenly in mid-movement. How are you standing? Is your posture good? Or are your shoulders hunched and is your abdomen protruding? Going through the movements in slow motion is another way of keeping a check on your posture.

Exercises at the Wall and in the Middle of the Pool

Most of the basic exercises and some of the special ones are performed at the pool wall where you can hold on securely to the rail. Later you should try moving to the middle of the pool where you can do the exercises without support. There are lots of possibilities for varying these exercises by bouncing, hopping or jumping. To keep your balance in the pool you have to follow the rhythm of the movement with your arms too.

Leg Circling (Standing Position)

Special Exercise 1:
1. Stand with the pool wall to your right and hold onto the rail. Keeping your right leg straight, raise your left leg slightly in front of you.
2. Draw a big circle in front of you with your left leg, swinging it in a clockwise direction up towards the surface of the pool and back down again. Repeat, this time counterclockwise.
3. Relax, turn round and repeat the exercise with the other leg.
4. It's up to you how often you repeat these exercises (or any of the other special exercises). You can decide for yourself how many you will do leisurely, how many energetically and how many rapidly.

Note:
You can be quite elastic when you're doing this exercise. When you swing your leg up, make an extra little circle when you reach the surface of the water. This will increase the effectiveness of the exercise and give your abdomen an extra workout.

Benefits:
This exercise has a noticeable effect on the thighs, abdomen and waist.

Special Exercise 2:
1. Stand with the pool wall on your right and hold onto the rail. Keeping your right leg straight, stretch your left leg out slightly towards the side.

2. Draw a large circle sideways with your leg, first clockwise, then counterclockwise.
3. Relax, turn round and repeat the exercise with the other leg. Repeat as often as you want.

Benefits:
Good for the hips and waist.

Special Exercise 3:
1. Stand with the pool wall to your right and hold onto the rail. Keeping your right leg straight, stretch your left leg out slightly behind you.
2. Make a large circle behind you with your left leg, first clockwise, then counterclockwise.
3. Relax, turn round and repeat the same exercise with the other leg.

Note:
This is the most difficult leg-circling movement, but with practice you can master it.

Benefits:
Good for your buttocks and back.

Leg Circling (While Floating on Your Back)

Special Exercise:
1. Lie on your back in the water, hold onto the rail with both hands and stretch your legs, keeping them apart.
2. Make circles with both your legs at once—first outwards and then inwards. Your abdomen will move automatically with the rhythm of this exercise.

3. When you've finished the circling, shake your legs and kick them vigorously in the water.

Variations:
1. Gradually increase the size of the circles you make. The illustration shows how you can use the corner of the pool for this. (See Illus. 29.)

Illus. 29

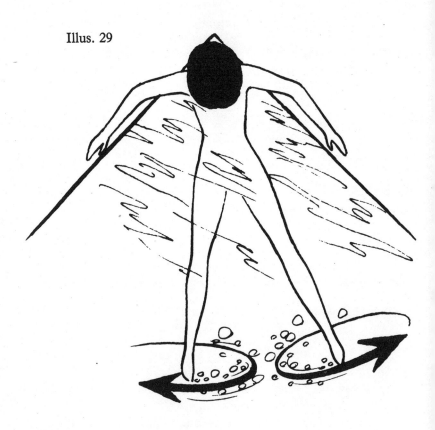

2. Emphasize the movement of your abdomen as you do the exercise.

3. Try the exercise in other positions; e.g., on your stomach at the rail or on your stomach in the corner of the pool.

Benefits:
Depending on the energy with which you practice the various positions in the water, this exercise works on the abdomen, hips and waistline. If you try this same exercise resting on your stomach, it will work on the hips, buttocks and back.

Figure Eights

Special Exercise:
1. Stand sideways to the wall and hold onto the rail with one hand. Stand on the leg closest to the wall and raise your other leg diagonally across your body.
2. Swing your free leg in a large "Figure Eight" in front of you.
3. The "Figure Eight" exercise can be done in all the same variations as the leg-circling exercises. That way you involve your entire body in the movements. (See Illus. 30.)

Variations:
1. Bounce a little on your supporting leg so you can make even larger Eights.
2. Include your abdomen in the "Figure Eight" movements.

Benefits:
This exercise improves the stomach, hips, thighs and buttocks.

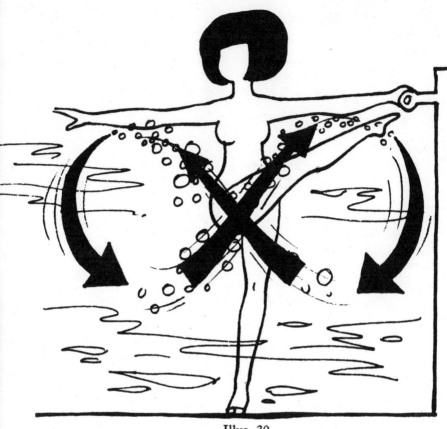

Illus. 30

Floating Eights

Warm-Up:
1. Face the side of the pool and grasp the handrail with both hands. Stand on the tips of your toes.
2. Extend your right leg slightly and trace a circle with your foot on the bottom of the pool.
3. As soon as you return to the starting position, repeat the same

movement with the other leg. The two circles you have made form a "Figure Eight."

Special Exercise:
1. Assume the same starting position as for warm-up 1.
2. Now make a "Figure Eight" with both legs, circling them both at the same time. Your feet don't touch the bottom of the pool this time.

Variations:
1. Let your abdomen follow the movements of your legs.
2. Turn your abdomen deliberately in the direction of each movement.

Benefits:
This special exercise increases the flexibility of your abdomen and waist.

Bent Circles and Figure Eights

Special Exercise:
1. Repeat all the circling and "Figure Eight" movements, but this time don't keep your legs straight.
2. Now trace all the circles and "Figure Eights" with your knee. Starting position is the same as in previous exercises.

Variations:
1. The resistance of the water is greatly reduced when you do this exercise, so you should increase the tempo.

2. Turn your abdomen more energetically in the direction of the exercise.
3. Repeat the exercises, changing back and forth from straight-legged figures to bent-legged figures.

Benefits:
This exercise is directed at the abdomen, hips and buttocks.

Arm Circling and Figure Eights

Special Exercise:
1. Standing on the tips of your toes in the middle of the pool, use your arms to make circles and "Figure Eights." (See Illus. 31.)
2. Do the exercise with your arms held straight and then with your arms bent. This time it's not your abdomen but your shoulders that are included.

Note:
Your arms and shoulders should be under the water during this exercise. Put more energy into the *backwards* swing of your arms.

Benefits:
Your arms and shoulders get a good workout in this exercise.

Variation 1:
1. Stand on your tiptoes in the middle of the pool, legs apart.
2. Stretch your arms out in front of you at shoulder height. Swing them down together past the sides of your body and out behind you as far as you can. Swing back again the same way to starting position.

Benefits:
The aim of this exercise is to give you a slimmer, more flexible upper body. The water massages your shoulders and arms.

Variation 2:

1. Repeat the same exercise as described in Variation 1, but swing one of your legs back as you swing your arms forwards again.

Benefits:

Increases the effect of this exercise on your buttocks and back.

Variation 3:

1. Stand in the middle of the pool on your tiptoes, feet slightly apart.
2. Swing your arms freely back and forth and at the same time either walk or jump along the pool bottom. Go all the way across the pool this way.

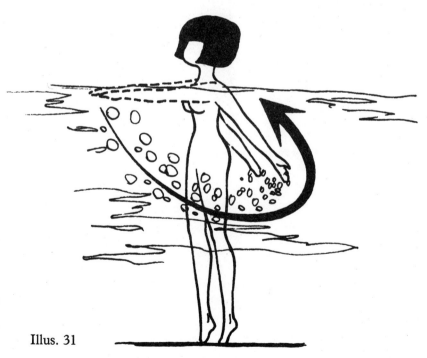

Illus. 31

Circles Galore

Now that you've traced circles and "Figure Eights" with your arms and legs, it's time to do them with other parts of your body too:
1. With hands and forearms.
2. With ankles and lower legs. (See Illus. 32.)
3. With your abdomen and with your upper body.

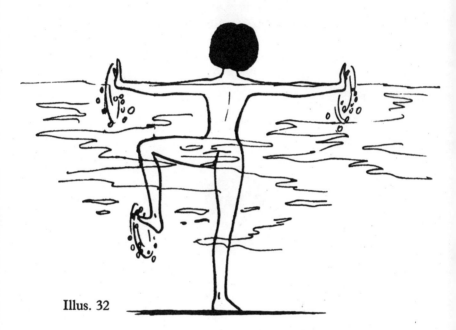

Illus. 32

The Flipper

Special Exercise:

1. Stand in the middle of the pool, legs slightly apart. Raise arms to shoulder height and bend your elbows so your hands touch each other, palms down, in front of your chest. Arms and shoulders should be underwater.

2. Now flap your elbows up and down very quickly. Put more energy into the downwards movement to begin with, then stress the upwards movement. (See Illus. 33.)

Variations:
1. Gradually increase the speed of your flapping movements.
2. Let your body move forwards with the upwards movement of your arms.
3. Give a little jump with each upwards and downwards movement of your arms.

Benefits:
Pushing downwards with your elbows provides a good massage for your arms and chest.
Pushing upwards directly affects the fatty areas of your neck.
Both the upwards and downwards movements help to make your shoulders more flexible.

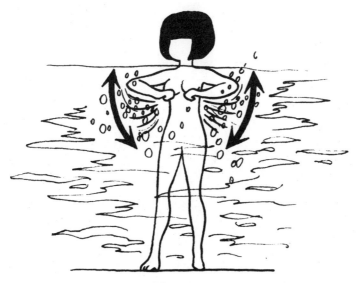

Illus. 33

Fluttering

Special Exercise:

1. Stand on your tiptoes in the middle of the pool. Extend your arms sideways at shoulder height, keeping your hands relaxed.
2. Flutter up and down with your arms, like a bird when it learns to fly. Your arms should go all the way down to your sides each time. (See Illus. 34.)
3. Turn the palms of your hands upwards and repeat the fluttering movements.
4. Turn your palms up for each upwards movement, down for each downwards movement. Flutter your way across the pool this way.

Benefits:

This exercise is aimed at slimming arms and chest and at giving your shoulders more flexibility.

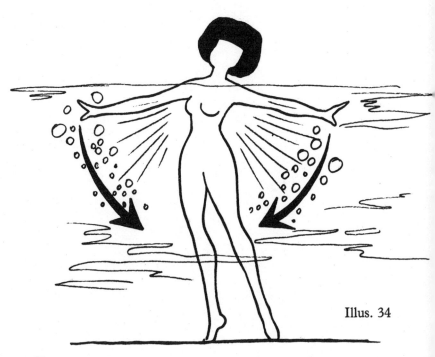

Illus. 34

Flip and Flutter

Special Exercise:
1. Stand in the middle of the pool, legs apart, arms at shoulder height, elbows bent and hands touching across your chest (as for the "Flipper"—see page 62).
2. Now stretch your arms out in front of you and swing them round and as far behind you as possible, keeping them at shoulder height.
3. Pull your arms back round in front of you and return to your starting position. Repeat the whole exercise.

Note:
At the end of your backwards swing, give your arms an extra little pull as though you were trying to make them touch, before you swing them back to starting position.

Benefits:
This exercise will help you achieve straight, slender shoulders and slimmer arms.

Variation 1:
To benefit your back and buttocks as well, stretch your left and right leg alternately behind you as you do this exercise.

Variation 2:
Now combine the movements from the special exercise and Variation 1. This will result in a kind of "walking swim."
Keep your legs fairly stiff and don't bother giving your arms that extra bounce. Alternate your left and right leg and keep your backwards swing quite forceful.

Benefits:
Good for your entire body.

Variation 3:
Legs apart, stand on your tiptoes and lean forwards with your entire body, making sure you don't bend at the waist. Use the arm movement you've just learned to keep your balance.

Benefits:
Good for posture and especially effective for your arms and shoulders.

The Little Angel

Special Exercise:
1. Stand facing the wall of the pool. Stretch both arms wide and hold onto the rail with both hands. Keep your feet apart. You should stand as far away from the wall as you can.
2. Bend you arms and push your chest forwards till it touches the pool wall. Go onto your toes as you do this.

Variation 1:
Stretch first one leg and then the other out behind you as you do this exercise.

Benefits:
Helps make chest and shoulders slender and supple.

Variation 2:
Change the position of your hands and legs. Swing your body towards one hand and then towards the other, instead of straight towards the wall.

Benefits:
Helps make chest and pelvis flexible.

Special Exercise:
1. Face the pool wall, spread your arms out wide and grasp the rail with your hands. Stand with your feet apart. Now swing your

upper body from one side to the other, parallel to the wall, shifting your weight as you do so.

2. Now repeat the movement, swinging your upper body round as far as possible—so far in each direction, in fact, that you're forced to take one foot off the bottom each time.

Variation 1:
Repeat the same movements, this time letting your abdomen perform the swinging movements instead of your upper body. (See Illus. 35.)

Variation 2:
Swing your entire body (chest and abdomen together) from one side to the other.

Benefits:
This exercise helps give you a supple body and good posture.

Illus. 35

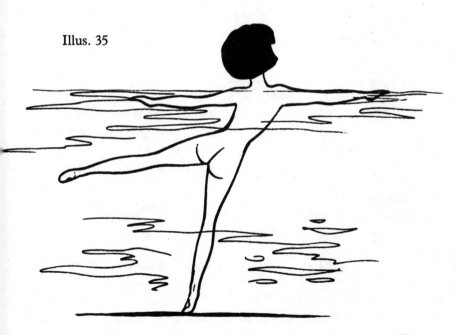

Push and Swing

Special Exercise:
1. Stand with some distance between you and the pool wall. Face the edge of the pool and grasp the rail with both hands. Your legs should be together and your body slightly inclined.
2. Bending your arms, let your body drop quickly forwards towards the wall. Then push back to starting position by straightening your arms.

Note:
The faster you do this exercise, the greater the massage effect it will have.

Benefits:
Your whole body (especially your waist and hips) gets a good massage from the water.

Variation:
1. Place both feet together on the wall.
2. With quick movements, bend and straighten your legs. If there are steps you can use, try doing this exercise on each step, one after the other.

Benefits:
Your upper thighs, particularly, get a good massage from this exercise.

The "Swing" seems to develop naturally from this exercise.

Special Exercise:
1. Place both feet together on the wall.

2. Now swing your abdomen backwards and forwards. Your arms and legs will straighten automatically.

Benefits:
Massages waist and back and increases flexibility.

Variation:
This time don't just swing your abdomen back and forth—move it in a circular motion.

The Stork Walk and the Stork Leap

Warm-Up:
1. Rest your arms on the water at shoulder height.
2. Keeping one leg straight, raise your other knee as high as you can, straighten your leg out and then lower it slowly back to the starting position.
3. Repeat this exercise as often as you like, varying the direction.

Benefits:
This exercise helps you with your sense of balance.

Special Exercise:
1. Start from the same basic position as the warm-up.
2. Raise your knee, straightening out your leg at the same time and transferring your weight forwards. Now you're doing the "Stork Walk." You can add to your momentum by making a swimming movement with your arms.

Benefits:
This exercise helps you achieve a good sense of balance as well as a good posture.
From this movement it's an easy transition to the "Stork Leap."

Special Exercise:
1. Start from the same position as for the warm-up.
2. This time push off strongly from the starting position with the leg you're standing on. Now you're leaping forwards with each move instead of just stepping. (See Illus. 36.)

Benefits:
The "Stork Leap" benefits your entire body.

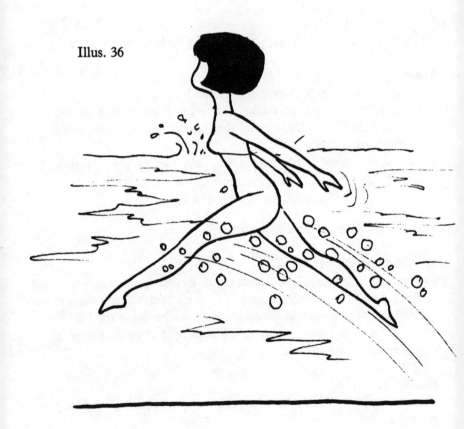

Illus. 36

The Figurehead

Special Exercise:
1. Stand in the pool with feet slightly apart.
2. Clasp your hands behind your back, arms straight.
3. Stretch your arms behind your back and pull your shoulders back at the same time.
4. Go up on your tiptoes and stretch your entire body.

Benefits:
Helps eliminate fatty deposits on your neck as well as round shoulders. This exercise is also good for your posture in general.

Variations:
1. Keep your legs together. (See Illus. 37.)

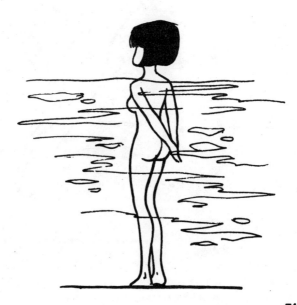

Illus. 37

2. Move your arms the way you did in the previous exercise.
3. As you stretch your arms and legs, lean forwards with your whole body and make a little jump to straighten up. (See Illus. 38.)

Note:
Repeat both exercises quickly, one after the other.

Benefits:
This exercise is good for the shoulders, chest and posture in general.

Illus. 38

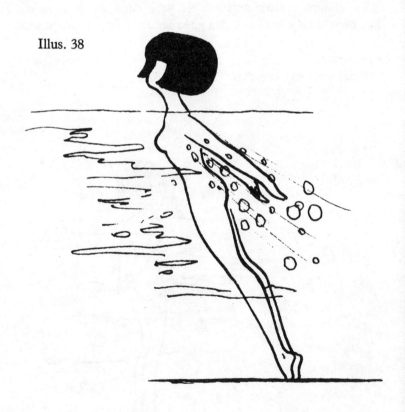

Along the Wall

Special Exercise:

1. Face the side of the pool and grasp the rail with both hands. With legs apart, put your feet up on the wall.
2. Now move your feet up and down the wall. Bounce away from the wall a little each time you change your foot position. (See Illus. 39.)
3. Relax and shake your legs.

Benefits:

This exercise is good for the flexibility of your legs in general.

Variations:

Turn round and do the same exercise, this time with your heels against the wall. Then give your legs a good shake.

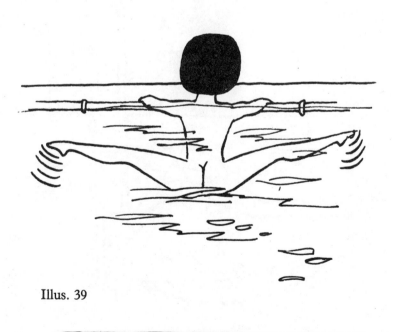

Illus. 39

The Pendulum

Special Exercise:
1. Face the wall and grasp the rail.
2. Place the foot of one leg against the wall and bend your knee. Bounce back and forth using your knee (i.e. keeping your foot on the wall).
3. Keep your other leg straight and swing it back and forth like a pendulum. This exercise can be done at the ladder as well as at the rail. (See Illus. 40.)
4. Repeat the exercise with the other leg.

Illus. 40

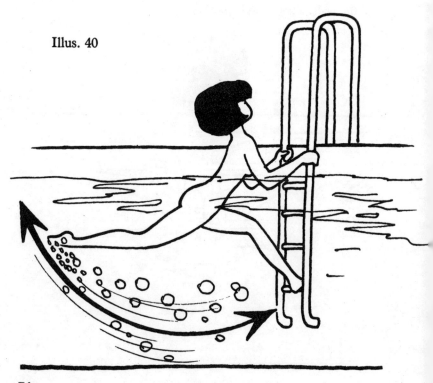

Variation:
Swing both legs together like a pendulum. (See Illus. 41.)

Note:
As you swing your "pendulum" leg back towards the wall, put so much energy into the swing that your other leg is forced to straighten out.

Benefits:
This exercise benefits buttocks and back and helps to increase overall flexibility.

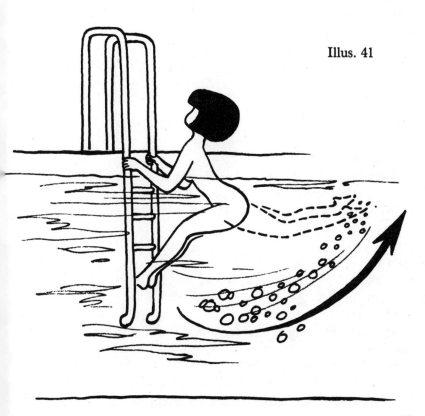

Illus. 41

The Big Kick

Special Exercise:
1. Face the wall of the pool and hold onto the rail with both hands.
2. Bend the knee of one leg and put your foot on the wall.
3. Put your other knee up to your chest and then kick out behind you with that same leg as energetically as you can. Swing your leg forwards again and bring your knee back up to your chest. (See Illus. 42.)

Benefits:
Stomach, buttocks, back, thighs and waist all benefit from this exercise.

The Bell

Special Exercise:
1. Face the wall of the pool, both hands on the rail.
2. Push off strongly from the wall with both feet.
3. Now swing both legs back and forth like a bell clapper, without touching the wall. (See Illus. 43.)

Benefits:
This exercise contributes to a slender, flexible waist.

Variation:
On the forward swing of your legs, bend your knees and bring them up to your chest.

Benefits:
This exercise is especially good for the stomach.

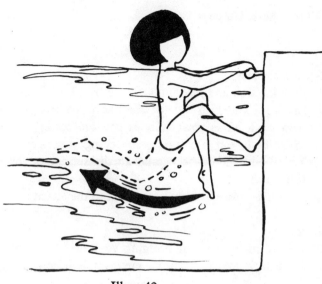

Illus. 42

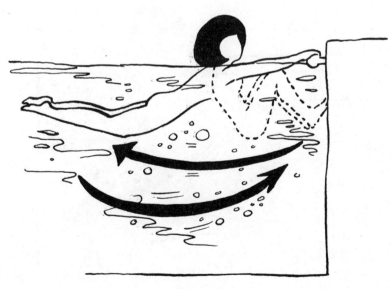

Illus. 43

The Big Wave

Special Exercise:
1. Face the wall and hold onto the rail with both hands.
2. Lift both knees up to your chest and put both feet on the wall.
3. Now push off as powerfully as you can so that you swing your entire body out backwards, stretching your legs as you do so. Your body should be parallel to the surface of the water. (See Illus. 44.)
4. Then let yourself drop slowly back to the starting position.

Note:
There are many ways of bringing your body back to the starting position once you've reached your maximum body swing.

Illus. 44

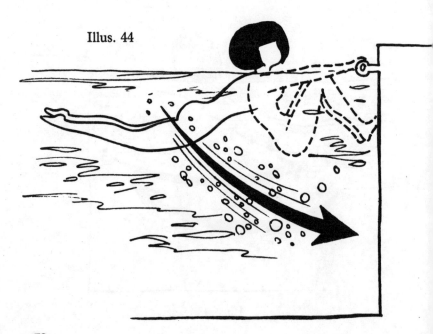

Variations:

1. Swing your body back towards the wall, abdomen first. Don't arch your back as you do this.
2. Turn your lower body first to the left and then to the right as you swing back. Do this slowly at first and then speed up. This quick movement is very effective for buttocks and abdomen.
3. Make circles with your legs in opposite directions as you swing back, first outwards and then inwards.

Benefits:
Helps your whole body become supple and slender.

Horizontal

Special Exercise:

1. Stand with the pool wall to your left and hold onto the rail with your left hand. Keep your left leg straight.
2. Raise your right leg slowly behind you and, going up on the tiptoes of your left foot, lean your upper body forwards, at the same time raising your right arm straight out in front of you. Your arm and leg should form a horizontal line.
3. Hold this position for a while and check your posture.
4. Try the same thing backwards. This exercise is quite a bit more difficult. Stretch your leg out in front of you and your arm out behind you.

Benefits:
This exercise makes your whole body feel good and has an improving effect on your posture.

Variation 1:
Alternate quickly from leg forwards to leg backwards. Let your supporting leg give slightly at the knee with each swing of the other leg. Hold each position for a moment before you change direction.

Variation 2:

1. Now try the same exercise in the middle of the pool. For better balance, stretch your arm out in front of you in the water. If you're doing the exercise with your right leg, then use your left arm for balance. (See Illus. 45.)
2. Once you've reached the "horizontal" position, take a little jump forwards.

Variation 3:

Having reached the "horizontal" position, with your left leg out in front of you and using your right leg as the supporting leg, jump

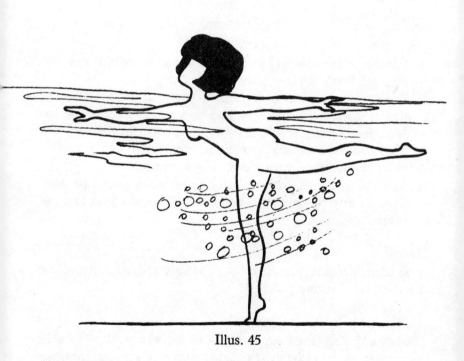

Illus. 45

lightly on the bottom of the pool and tilt your body backwards.
Return to the starting position again. (See Illus. 46.)

Benefits:
These exercises will help you to improve both your posture and
your balance.

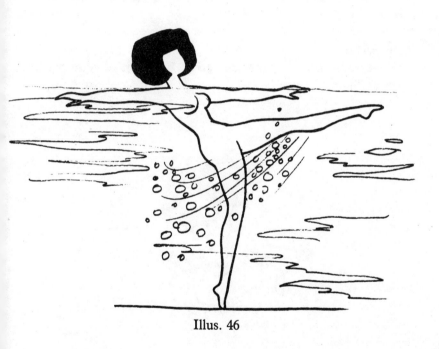

Illus. 46

The Locomotive

Special Exercise:
1. Stand in the middle of the pool. Raise your knees one after the other as high as you can and as strongly as you can.
2. At the same time bend your arms close to your sides, clench your fists and pump your arms back and forth like a child imitating a steam engine. (See Illus. 47.)

Note:
You can either do this exercise on the spot or you can move forwards as you do it.

Benefits:
This exercise affects your whole body. Every bit of extra padding gets a good massage.

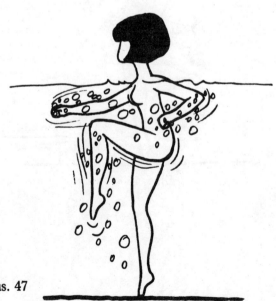

Illus. 47

The Water Snake

Special Exercise:
1. Lie on your back in the water, feet apart.
2. Twist your abdomen quickly from side to side, paddling with your forearms and hands at the same time.
3. You will move backwards through the water like a snake. (See Illus. 48.)

Variations:
1. To increase the twisting motion of your abdomen, pull your knees up as far as you can with each twist. At the same time, paddle more energetically with your hands.
2. Now pull up both knees and twist your entire lower body quickly from side to side.

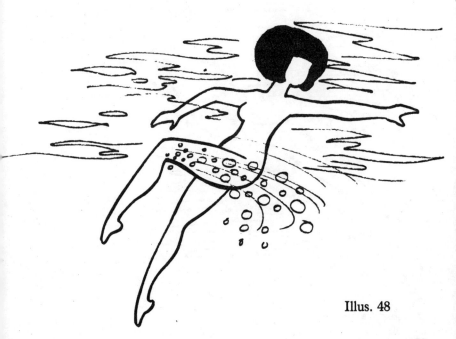

Illus. 48

3. To counterbalance the swing of your abdomen, let one arm stretch out behind you. For a right twist, the left arm will be behind, and vice versa. The other arm is bent towards your knees.
4. Do the same exercise, this time on your stomach. (See Illus. 49.)

Benefits:
This exercise provides your body with a very effective massage that is good for all your problem areas. It also helps make your arms and legs more flexible.

Illus. 49

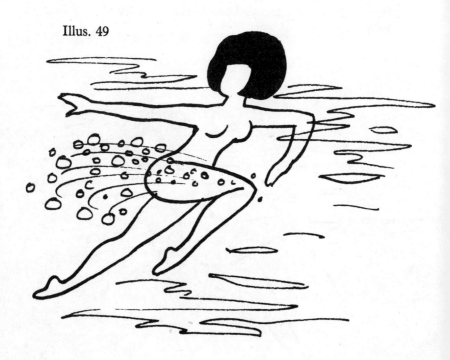

The Twist

We've already seen how the "Snake" (see page 83) is an excellent way of getting rid of unwanted fat. Now we can do this same motion all the way across the pool.

Special Exercise:
1. Stand on your toes, legs slightly bent.
2. Rest your arms on the water at shoulder height. They should also be slightly bent. (See Illus. 50.)
3. Twist your abdomen as quickly as possible from one side to the other.

Illus. 50

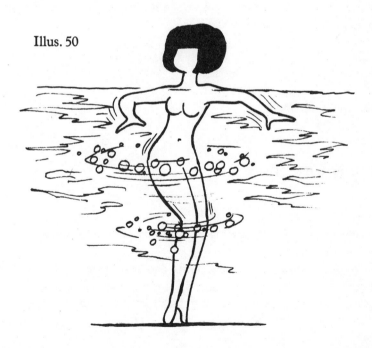

4. Put a lot of energy into the forward twist and lift your toes slightly off the bottom.
5. Paddle with your arms in the opposite direction of your body twist—and "twist" all the way across the pool.

Variation 1:
This time extend one leg slightly to the side and twist in the opposite direction.

Variation 2:
Now continue the same twisting movement, this time with one knee raised. Swing the dangling part of your leg back and forth in front of your body as you twist. Your arms supply the countermovements, so you can keep your balance.

Benefits:
This is one of the most popular exercises. It gets every fatty cell in your body moving.

Jumping Jack

Special Exercise:
1. Stand in the pool, legs together and arms at your sides.
2. Now jump energetically.
3. As you jump, spread your arms and legs wide, bend them in again and then stretch widely once more. (See Illus. 51.)
4. You can repeat the "Jumping Jack" in various directions.

Benefits:
This exercise is not very easy, but it's very good for taking off all your unwanted fat.

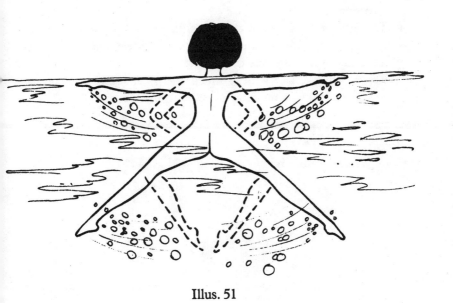

Illus. 51

Spinning Top

A top always needs some energy to get it spinning. Your slim, active, flexible body can supply the energy you need for this exercise.

Special Exercise:
1. Stand in the middle of the pool, legs together, arms resting lightly on the surface of the water.
2. Jump energetically, pushing yourself off the pool bottom quite forcefully.

3. As you jump, pull up your knees and twist both legs in one direction. At the same time, swing both arms in the opposite direction. (See Illus. 52.)
4. These movements will make you spin like a top in the water.
5. Let the motion end naturally and then repeat the movements, this time in the opposite direction.
6. Repeat this exercise with as much energy and speed as you can so you will spin as much as possible in the water.

Benefits:
Good for your entire body.

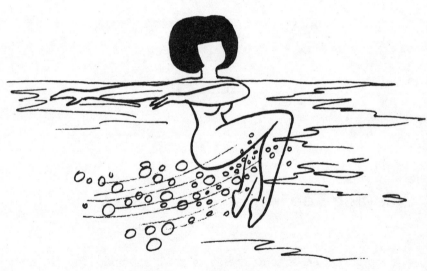

Illus. 52

The Thriller

The "Thriller" is the ultimate "Figure Eight" movement.

Special Exercise:
1. Face the pool wall and hold onto the rail with both hands.
2. Raise both knees, legs together, and put your feet on the pool wall.
3. Push off energetically from the wall and swing your entire body in a large "Figure Eight." Keep your legs straight and let your abdomen follow the motion of your legs.

Variation:
Repeat the exercise, using the pool ladder. (See Illus. 53.)

Benefits:
Good for your entire body.

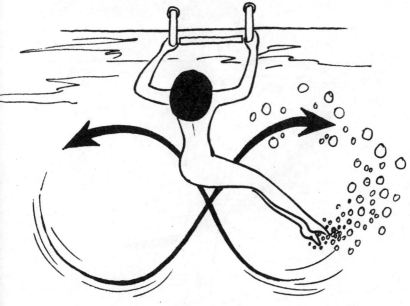

Illus. 53

The Big Bell

There is only one exercise left to master. The "Big Bell" gives you a real opportunity to test what condition your body is in and it should be included in all your Aqua-Rhythmic sessions.

Special Exercise:
1. Stand in the pool, legs together, arms outstretched in front of you.
2. Push off energetically from the pool bottom and swing both legs forwards, keeping them together.
3. Bend the upper part of your body forwards so you can touch your toes with your fingertips (the "Jack-Knife!").
4. Now swing your legs out behind you, still keeping them together. Paddle with your arms to help you swing back and forth like a bell. (See Illus. 54 and 55.)
5. Repeat this exercise ten times without stopping.

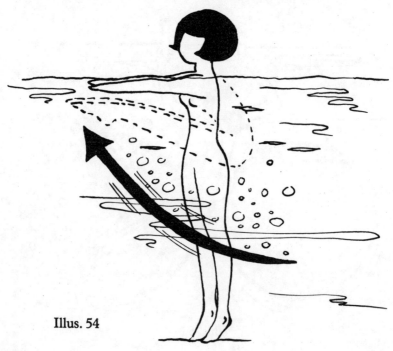

Illus. 54

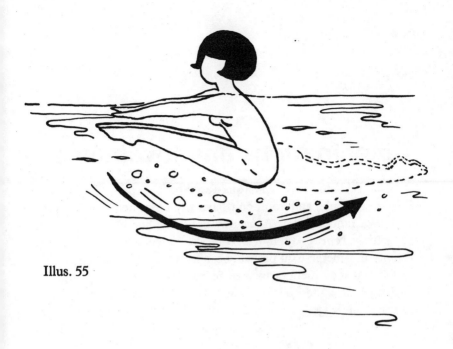

Illus. 55

Benefits:
Once you have mastered this exercise you have real reason to be proud of yourself. You've lost almost all your unwanted fat and when you leave the pool you'll feel lighter in every sense of the word.

Combinations and Inventions

Now you, too, are an Aqua-Rhythmics expert. You're slim, lithe and supple, and you don't have any unwanted fat to interfere with your mobility. The Aqua-Rhythmics method isn't simply a way of getting your body moving—it also increases your desire for activity in general. You probably can't wait to free your imagination and invent movements which correspond to your own rhythms and enable you to explore all your new potential. It's a glorious experience to reach this stage—and you have an added pleasure in knowing that all your activity has achieved something—your lovely, slender figure. You should keep a critical eye on your shape so you don't give unwanted fat a chance to accumulate.

Now your body reflects the way you feel and there are no limits to the types or combinations of movements you can do. You can also choose the rhythms that suit you best. Make use of every opportunity to test your flexibility. Invent as many new variations as you can!

How to Keep Your Good Figure

If you want to test whether Aqua-Rhythmics have helped you to achieve your goal of a good figure, then you should consult your mirror rather than your scales. Your mirror shows you where you've lost weight, but it also reflects your new proportions, your new muscle tone and your excellent posture. When you have a lithe and active body it shines through your whole appearance.

Aqua-Rhythmics have helped you to become elastic, healthy and lively because they demand a harmony of body and mind. This harmony is a source of pleasure as well as activity and is decisive for your new life-style. And that new life-style is what will enable you to keep your good figure. Now you realize that it's not difficult to quietly refuse certain foods and drinks that are not good for you and to eat proper, nourishing meals. It doesn't demand a sacrifice anymore to keep yourself trim. On the contrary—now that you're slim and supple you can really enjoy all the things you do to stay that way.

Aqua-Rhythmics will help you stay slim and hold onto that beautiful figure of yours!

Index

abdomen
  effect on posture, 53
  exercises, 25, 26, 34, 40, 41,
    42, 44, 47, 48, 49, 52, 54,
    57, 59
Along the Wall, 73
ankles, exercises, 26
appearance, personal, 10–11
Aqua-Rhythmics
  benefits, 8, 10, 15–16, 50
  innovation, 8
  strategy, 10, 19–20
Aqua-Rhythmics: Where and
  How?, 17–18
Arm Circling and Figure
  Eights, 60–61
arms, exercises, 36, 44, 49,
  60, 63, 64, 65, 66, 84
Arrangement of the Exercises,
  21–22
back, exercises, 33, 40, 41, 52,
  55, 57, 60, 65, 69, 75, 76
backwards movements, bene-
  fits, 52
balance exercises, 69, 81
Basic Principles of Aqua-
  Rhythmics, 19–20
Basic Regimen, 21, 23–49
Bell, 76–77
Bent Circles and Figure
  Eights, 59–60
Bicycle, 45–48
Big Bell, 90–91
Big Kick, 76–77
Big Wave, 78–79
blood circulation, 50
breathing, exercises, 36

buoyancy of water, 13
Butterfly Stroke, 35
buttocks, exercises, 25, 33, 40,
  41, 42, 48, 52, 55, 57, 60, 65
  75, 76
calves, exercises, 26, 47
cellulitis, 13
chest, exercises, 36, 63, 64,
  66, 72
Circles Galore, 62
circulation, 50
Combinations and Inventions,
  92
Dancer, 25, 31–33
deep breathing, 50
directional variations, 19–20,
  52
eating habits, 8
energetic mode, 20
exercises for
  abdomen, 25, 26, 34, 40,
    41, 42, 44, 47, 48, 49, 52,
    54, 57, 59
  ankles, 26
  arms, 36, 44, 49, 60, 63, 64,
    65, 66, 84
  back, 33, 40, 41, 52, 55, 57,
    60, 65, 69, 75, 76
  balance, 69, 81
  breathing, 36
  buttocks, 25, 33, 40, 41, 42,
    48, 52, 55, 57, 60, 65, 75,
    76
  calves, 26, 47
  chest, 36, 63, 64, 66, 72
  feet, 47
  hips, 25, 29, 40, 42, 48, 49,
    52, 55, 57, 68
  knees, 26

legs, 29, 40, 41, 44, 47, 49, 73, 84
neck, 63
pelvis, 66
posture, 66, 67, 69, 71, 72, 79, 81
shoulders, 36, 60, 63, 64, 65, 66, 72
stomach, 25, 34, 57, 76
thighs, 25, 26, 33, 40, 47, 49, 52, 54, 57, 68, 76
upper body, 60
waistline, 33, 42, 47, 48, 52, 54, 55, 57, 59, 68, 69, 76
whole body, 36, 44, 65, 67, 68, 70, 75, 79, 82, 84, 86, 88, 89, 91
Exercises at the Wall and in the Middle of the Pool, 53–54
fat spots, 21
feet, exercises, 47
Figure Eights, 57
figure
  ideal, 9–11
  maintaining, 93
Figurehead, 71–72
flexibility, 50
Flip and Flutter, 65–66
Flipper, 62–63
Floating Eights, 58–59
Fluttering, 64
forward movements, benefits, 52
Frog by the Wall, 29–30, 48
Frog in the Pool, 48–49
Frog Kick, 35
group exercises, 18
healing properties of water, 12

hip exercises, 25, 29, 40, 42, 48, 49, 52, 55, 57, 68
Horizontal, 79–81
How to Keep Your Good Figure, 93
Ideal Figure: A Big Problem, 9–11
Individual and the Group, 18
introduction, 7–8
invention of new movements, 92
Jack-Knife, 43–44
jumping exercises, 43–44
Jumping Jack, 86–87
Kicking, 24–25
knees, exercises, 26
"Knees Up," 25, 33
Kneipp, Pastor, 12
Leg Circling (Standing Position), 54–55
Leg Circling (While Floating on Your Back), 55–57
legs, exercises, 29, 40, 41, 44, 47, 49, 73, 84
leisurely mode, 20
life-styles, 9
Little Angel, 66–67
Locomotive, 82
lymphatic system, 50
massage, water, 13
mirror, use of, 10–11
movement variations, 19–20
neck, exercises, 63
non-swimmers, 15, 23, 36
nude exercising, 18
nutrition, 8
participants in Aqua-Rhythmics, 15–16
pelvis, exercises, 66
Pendulum, 74–75

Personal Introduction, 7–8
pool therapy, 12
Posture, 52, 53
   exercises, 66, 67, 69, 71,
     72, 79, 81
proportion, 52
Push and Swing, 68–69
Qualities of Water, 13–14
rapid mode, 20
reducing systems, 9–10
Refreshing Pause, 50–51
relaxing effects of Aqua-
   Rhythmics, 16
resistance, water, 13
rest period, 50–51
rhythm variations, 19–20
safeness of Aqua-Rhythmics, 15
scales, use of, 10–11
Scissors, 37–41, 46
security of water, 13
senior citizens, 13, 15
Shake, 41–42
shoulder, exercises, 36, 60,
   63, 64, 65, 66, 72
sidewards movements, benefits, 52
sitting posture, 53
sociability of Aqua-Rhythmics, 18
Special Regimen, 21–22, 52–91
speed, effects of, 25
Spinning Top, 87–88
stomach, exercises, 25, 34,
   57, 76
Stork Walk and Stork Leap,
   69–70
Superkick, 33–34
Swimming, 23
Swimming in Place, 34–36

Swimming Pool, 17–18
swimsuits, 18
Swing, 68–69
tempo, 52
thighs, exercises, 25, 26, 33,
   34, 40, 47, 49, 52, 54, 57,
   68, 76
Thriller, 89
thrust, effects of, 25
Treading Water, 25–28, 33
turning movements, benefits,
   52
Twist, 85–86
underwater movements, 8,
   12–14
upper body
   effect on posture, 53
   exercises, 60
variations, importance of, 19–
   20
Varying the Direction, 20
Varying the Movements, 20
Varying the Rhythm, 19–20
waist, exercises, 33, 42, 47,
   48, 52, 54, 55, 57, 59, 68,
   69, 76
walking swim, 65
Water and How It Can Help
   You, 12–14
Water Snake, 83–84, 85
weight-loss programs, 9–11
Who Can Do Aqua-Rhyth-
   mics, 15–16
whole-body exercises, 36, 44,
   65, 67, 68, 70, 75, 79, 82,
   84, 86, 88, 89, 91
With or Without a Swimsuit,
   18
workout time, 21